N.L. CASH

Strength from Yoga: Gentle Practices for Seniors

This book was professionally typeset on Reedsy.
Find out more at reedsy.com

Contents

1

Introduction to Yoga for Seniors

Welcome to "Strength From Yoga: Gentle Practices For Seniors: Ease of Yoga: Simple Practices for Senior Wellness." This book will explore the importance of maintaining physical fitness and mobility as we age. My parents are in the senior age group, and I'm frequently seeking health and wellness research to help them improve their quality of life. Fun fact: Did you know that according to the U.S. Census Bureau, there are approximately 62 million individuals aged 65 and older in the United States as of 2024? This demographic group accounted for about 16% of the total U.S. population. In 30 years, by 2054, there will be approximately 84 million individuals aged 65 and older in the U.S. This Staggering growth rate also indicates the importance of senior health and wellness platforms.

I'm thrilled to launch this book, "Strength From Yoga: Gentle Practices For Seniors: Ease of Yoga: Simple Practices for Senior Wellness," for which I have a great passion. You'll be pleased to hear that I will soon write additional books on Chair Exercises for Seniors and Basic Gentle Stretching for Seniors. Be on the lookout at Amazon for the following two books!

As individuals gracefully age, maintaining physical and mental well-being becomes paramount. With its ancient roots and holistic approach, yoga emerges as a powerful tool for seniors seeking a path to health and vitality. In this chapter, we introduce yoga for seniors, exploring its origins, principles, and the tailored benefits it offers this demographic.

Understanding the Essence of Yoga

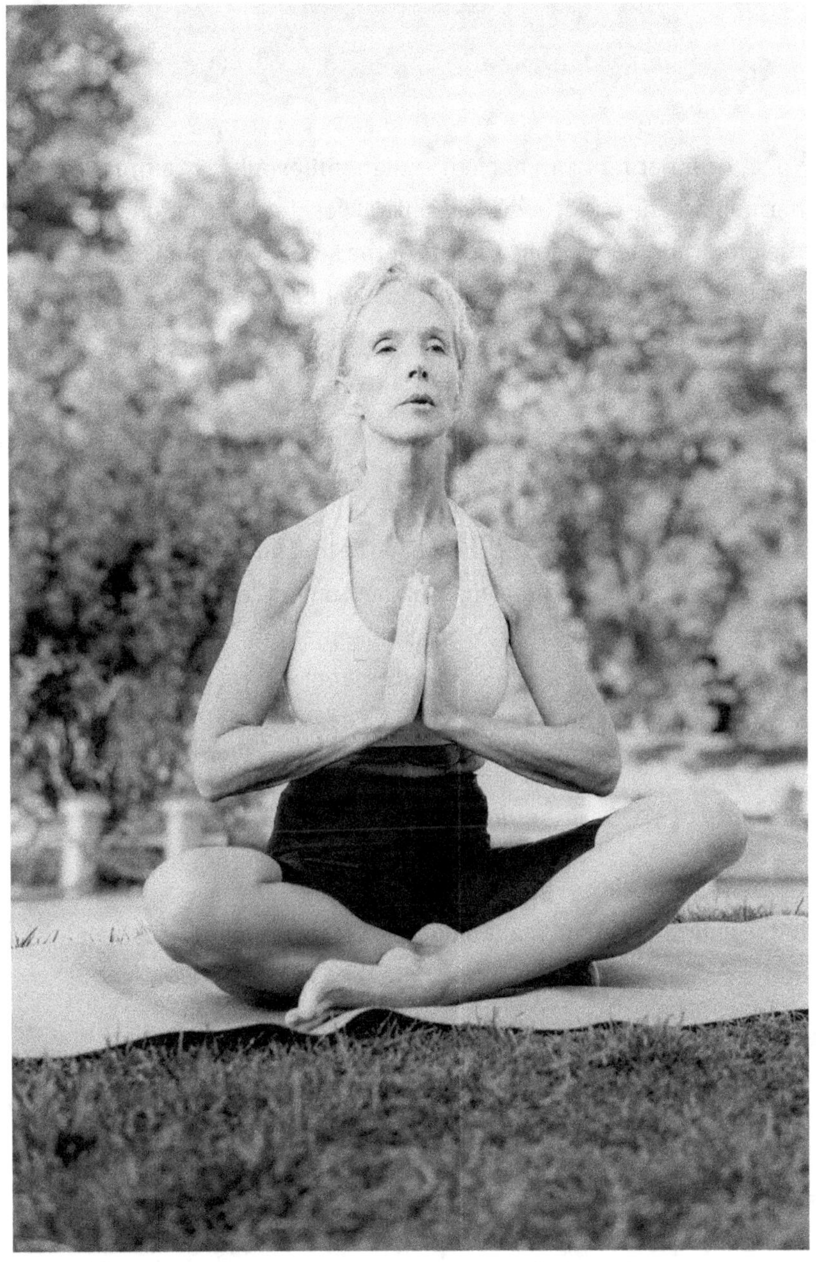

Yoga, originating from ancient Indian philosophy, is a practice that harmonizes the mind, body, and spirit. "yoga" means union, signifying the integration of various aspects of the self. It encompasses physical postures (asanas), breath control (pranayama), meditation, and ethical principles that guide one's conduct and lifestyle.

Tailored Yoga for Seniors

Yoga for seniors is a modified approach that embraces traditional yoga principles while considering the unique needs and limitations associated with aging. This adaptation ensures that seniors can reap the numerous benefits of yoga in a safe and accessible manner. Gentle movements, emphasis on breath awareness, and the integration of mindfulness make yoga ideal for seniors looking to enhance their overall quality of life.

Benefits of Yoga for Seniors

Improved Flexibility: Yoga's gentle stretches and poses enhance flexibility, aiding seniors in maintaining a full range of motion in their joints and muscles.

Enhanced Strength: The weight-bearing nature of many yoga poses helps build and maintain muscle strength, which is crucial for daily activities.

Balance and Stability: Yoga poses that focus on balance contribute to stability and reduce the risk of falls, a common concern for seniors.

Stress Reduction: Yoga's mindful breathing and meditation components promote relaxation, reduce stress, and contribute to mental well-being.

Joint Health: Yoga's low-impact nature is gentle on joints, making it an excellent choice for seniors managing conditions like arthritis.

Getting Started with Yoga

Embarking on a yoga journey doesn't require prior experience or extraordinary flexibility. Before trying yoga, my parents had zero yoga experience over the past 50 years. Seniors can start at their own pace, choosing classes or routines that cater specifically to their needs. Whether practicing at home or joining a local class, the key is consistency and embracing the process.

In the upcoming chapters, we will explore specific yoga poses, routines, and meditation techniques tailored for seniors. By embracing yoga, seniors can cultivate strength, flexibility, and balance, fostering a journey toward optimal health and vitality.

2

Understanding the Benefits of Yoga for Seniors

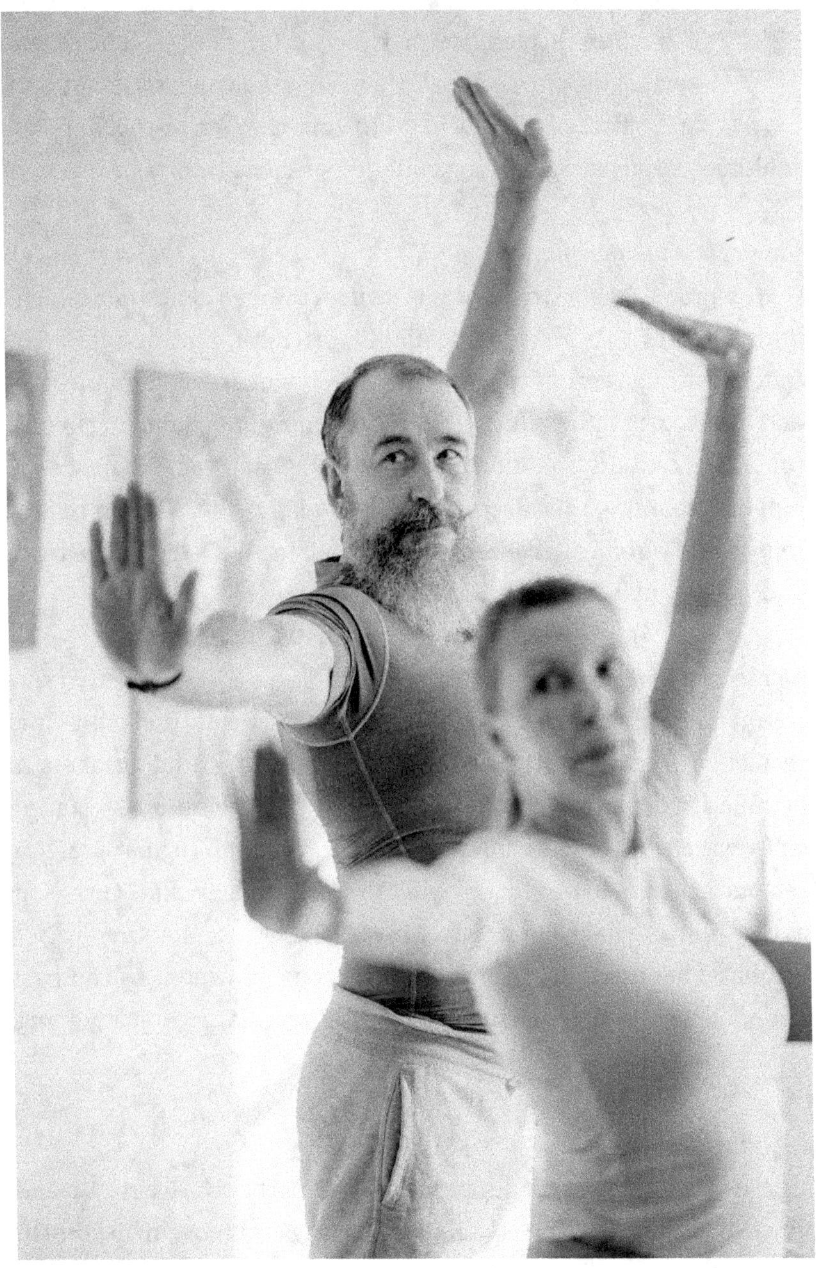

Yoga offers a plethora of benefits for seniors that extend beyond the physical realm, encompassing mental, emotional, and spiritual well-being. In this chapter, we explore the multifaceted advantages of yoga tailored specifically for seniors.

Physical Health Benefits:

Yoga promotes physical health in seniors through gentle movements and stretches that enhance flexibility, strength, and balance. The practice of yoga asanas (poses) helps seniors maintain joint mobility and muscle strength, reducing the risk of injury and improving overall functional capacity. Additionally, yoga poses that focus on balance can enhance stability, thus decreasing the likelihood of falls and related injuries—a significant concern for older adults. We'll dig into balance and stability in more detail in upcoming chapters.

Mental and Emotional Well-being:

Beyond its physical benefits, yoga cultivates mental and emotional resilience in seniors. Its mindful nature encourages practitioners to become attuned to their thoughts, emotions, and sensations, fostering self-awareness and emotional regulation. Through regular practice, seniors may experience reduced levels of stress, anxiety, and depression, as yoga promotes relaxation and a sense of inner peace. Moreover, yoga's emphasis on mindfulness and present-moment awareness can help seniors cope with the challenges and transitions that accompany aging, promoting a more positive outlook on life.

Cognitive Enhancement:

Research suggests that yoga may also support cognitive health and function in seniors. The combination of physical movement, breath awareness, and meditation in yoga practice stimulates brain activity and promotes neuroplasticity—the brain's ability to adapt and rewire itself.

By engaging in yoga regularly, seniors may experience improvements in cognitive function, memory, and attention span, thus enhancing overall cognitive well-being as they age.

Social Connection and Community:

Participating in yoga classes provides seniors with opportunities for social connection and community engagement, which are essential for overall well-being. Joining a yoga class fosters a sense of camaraderie and belonging, as seniors connect with like-minded individuals who share similar interests and goals. The supportive environment of a yoga community encourages seniors to stay committed to their practice and fosters a sense of accountability, promoting consistency and long-term adherence to yoga as a lifestyle choice. Get out and make some new yoga friends!

In summary, yoga offers a holistic approach to health and well-being for seniors, addressing physical, mental, emotional, and social aspects of wellness. By understanding the diverse benefits of yoga, seniors can embark on a positive journey toward optimal health and vitality in their later years.

3

Gentle Yoga Poses for Strength and Flexibility

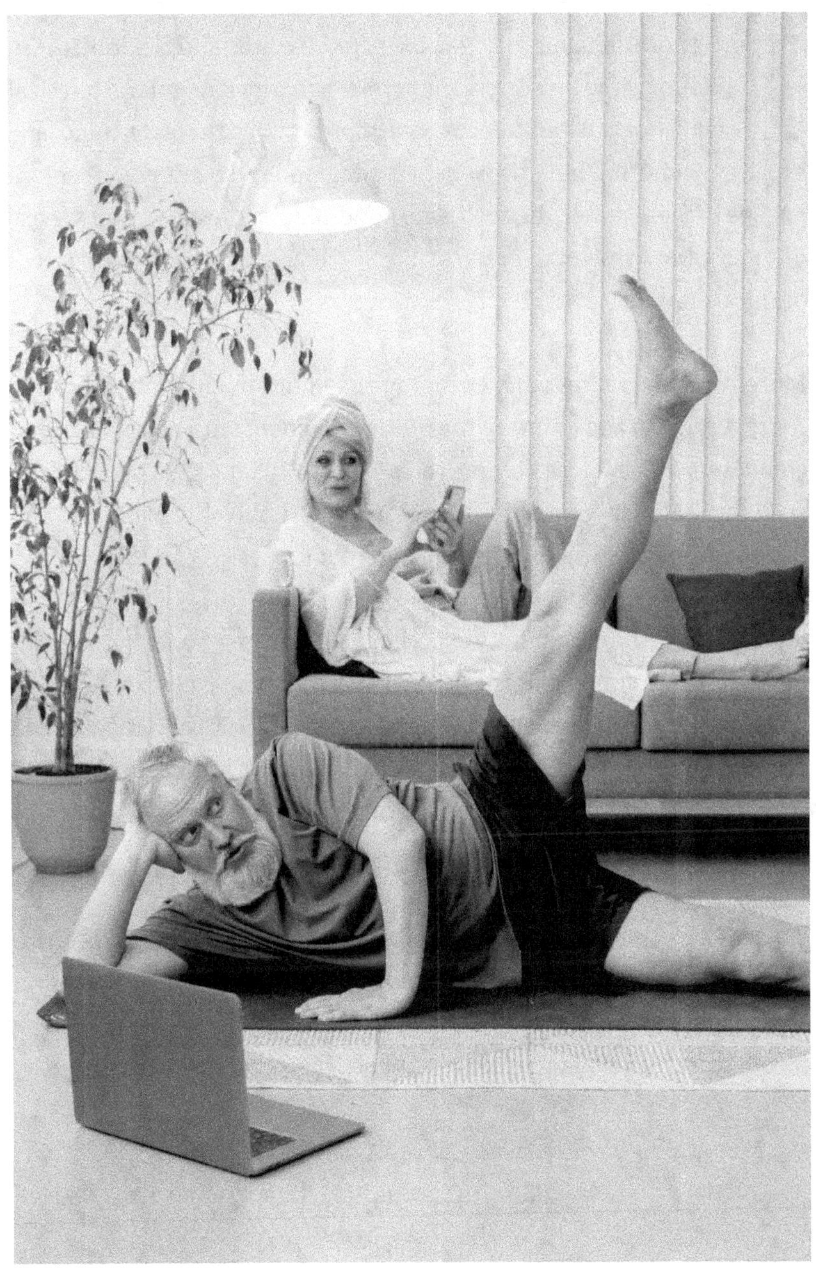

Incorporating gentle yoga poses for strength and flexibility into a senior's routine offers numerous benefits beyond the physical realm. Yoga fosters a deep connection between the body, mind, and breath, promoting holistic well-being and inner harmony. As seniors engage in these poses, they cultivate mindfulness, presence, and a sense of inner calm, which can be particularly valuable during times of stress or uncertainty.

Moreover, practicing yoga encourages seniors to cultivate gratitude for their bodies and embrace the present moment with acceptance and compassion. Each pose becomes an opportunity for self-discovery and self-care, allowing seniors to explore their bodies' capabilities and limitations with curiosity and non-judgment.

Furthermore, the community aspect of yoga can give seniors a sense of belonging and support as they embark on their yoga journey together. Sharing the practice with others fosters a sense of camaraderie and connection, enriching their overall yoga experience and deepening their appreciation for the positive power of gentle yoga poses. Feeling like you're making a difference for yourself and others is great.

Yoga offers a treasure trove of poses catering to seniors' needs, promoting strength and flexibility while honoring the body's limitations. In this chapter, we explore a selection of gentle yoga poses that seniors can incorporate into their practice to enhance physical well-being.

- **Mountain Pose (Tadasana)**:
- Begin by standing tall with feet hip-width apart and arms relaxed by your sides.
- Ground your feet into the earth and engage your thighs, lifting your kneecaps.

- Lengthen your spine, roll your shoulders back, and gently lift your chest.
- Mountain pose cultivates awareness of posture and alignment while promoting balance and stability.
- **Chair Pose (Utkatasana):**
- From mountain pose, inhale as you raise your arms overhead, palms facing each other.
- Exhale and bend your knees, lowering your hips as if sitting back in an imaginary chair.
- Keep your weight in your heels and your knees stacked over your ankles.
- Engage your core and lengthen your tailbone toward the floor.
- The chair pose strengthens the thighs, calves, and core muscles while improving balance and focus.
- **Tree Pose (Vrksasana):**
- Stand tall with feet rooted firmly into the ground.
- Shift your weight onto your left foot and lift your right foot off the ground, placing the sole against the inner left thigh or calf, avoiding the knee.
- Find your balance and bring your palms together at your heart center or extend your arms overhead.
- Tree pose builds leg strength and improves balance, stability, and concentration.
- **Warrior II (Virabhadrasana II):**
- Begin in a wide-legged stance, turning your right foot out 90 degrees and your left foot slightly inward.
- Bend your right knee over your right ankle, keeping your left leg straight.
- Extend your arms parallel to the ground, with your shoulders relaxed.
- Gaze over your right fingertips.

- Warrior II strengthens the legs, opens the hips, and cultivates stability and endurance.
- **Seated Forward Fold (Paschimottanasana):**
- Sit on the floor with your legs extended in front of you.
- Inhale to lengthen the spine, then exhale as you hinge at the hips and fold forward over your legs.
- Keep your back straight and reach for your feet or shins, resting your hands wherever feel comfortable.
- Seated forward fold stretches the spine, hamstrings, and lower back, promoting flexibility and relaxation.

As seniors explore these gentle yoga poses, it's essential to honor their bodies' limitations and practice with mindfulness and self-compassion. Please make sure that you're looking out for your safety. With regular practice, these poses can gradually enhance strength, flexibility, and overall well-being, supporting seniors on their journey to healthy aging through yoga.

4

Mindfulness and Meditation Practices for Seniors

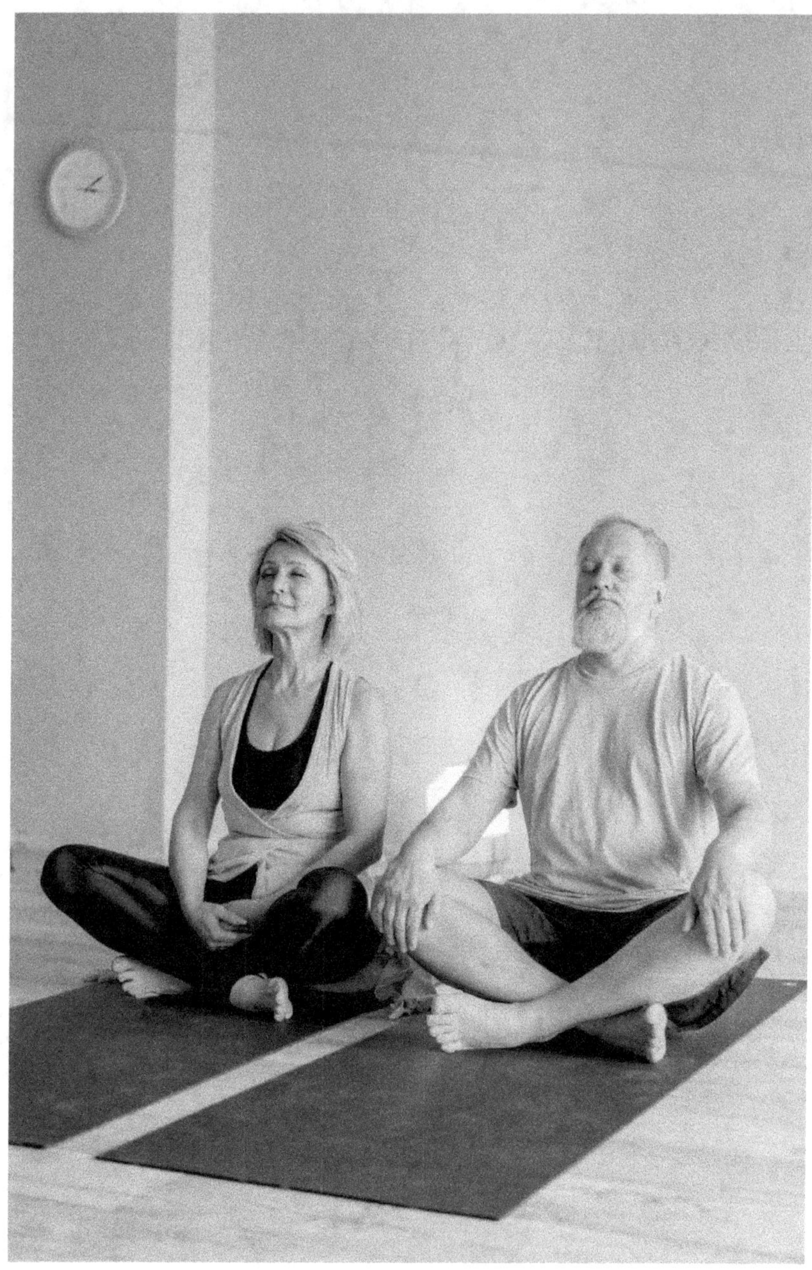

Mindfulness and meditation practices offer seniors powerful tools for cultivating inner peace, emotional resilience, and mental clarity. In this chapter, we explore how seniors can incorporate mindfulness and meditation into their daily lives to enhance overall well-being and quality of life.

Mindfulness involves paying attention to the present moment with openness, curiosity, and acceptance. It encourages seniors to bring their full awareness to their thoughts, emotions, bodily sensations, and surrounding environment without judgment. By practicing mindfulness, seniors can develop greater self-awareness, reduce stress, and cultivate a deeper sense of contentment and gratitude in their lives. Full mind, body, and emotional experience.

One simple mindfulness practice for seniors is **mindful breathing.**

- Seniors can find a quiet and comfortable place to sit or lie down and pay attention to the sensations of their breath as it moves in and out of their bodies.
- Focusing on the breath helps seniors anchor themselves in the present moment, letting go of worries about the past or future and experiencing a sense of calm and relaxation.

Another mindfulness practice that seniors can explore is **mindful walking.**

- This involves paying attention to each step as they walk slowly and deliberately, feeling the sensations of their feet making contact with the ground, and noticing the sights, sounds, and smells around them.
- Mindful walking can be done indoors or outdoors, allowing seniors

to connect with nature and appreciate the beauty of the world around them.

In addition to mindfulness, meditation practices can benefit seniors by promoting relaxation, reducing anxiety, and improving mental focus. Meditation involves training the mind to cultivate qualities like compassion, kindness, and equanimity through various techniques such as breath awareness, loving-kindness meditation, and body scan meditation.

Breath awareness meditation:

- This is a simple yet powerful practice in which seniors focus their attention on the sensations of their breath without trying to change them in any way.
- As thoughts or distractions arise, seniors gently redirect their focus back to the breath, cultivating a sense of calm and centeredness.

Loving-kindness meditation:

- Involves generating feelings of goodwill and compassion towards oneself and others.
- Seniors can silently repeat phrases such as "May I be happy, may I be healthy, may I be safe, may I live with ease" while visualizing sending love and kindness to themselves and those around them.

Body scan meditation:

- Involves systematically bringing awareness to different parts of the body, starting from the toes and gradually moving up to the head.
- Seniors can notice any sensations, tension, or areas of discomfort

in each part of the body and practice softening and relaxing those areas with each exhale.

By incorporating mindfulness and meditation practices into their daily routines, seniors can experience greater peace of mind, improved emotional well-being, and a deeper connection to themselves and the world around them. These practices offer invaluable tools for navigating the ups and downs of life with grace, resilience, and inner strength.

5

Yoga for Pain Management and Chronic Conditions

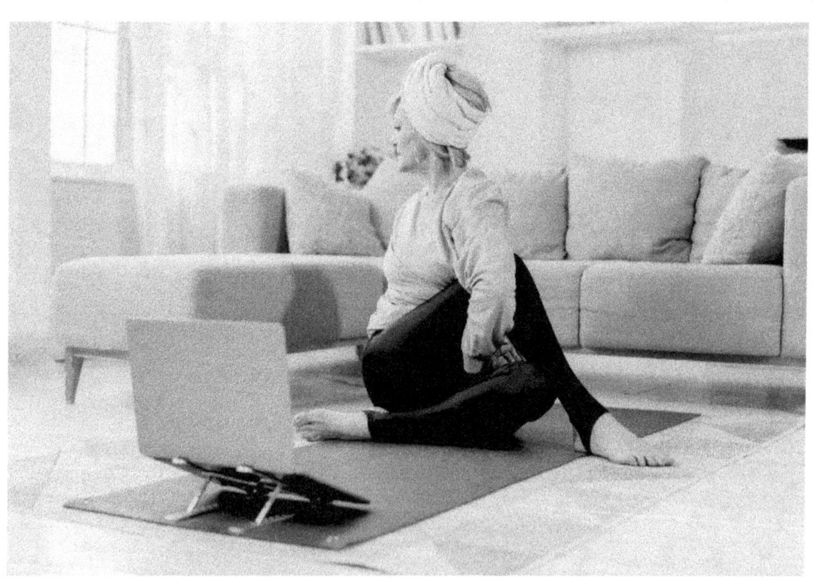

Yoga encourages seniors to listen to their bodies and honor their limitations, fostering a sense of self-compassion and acceptance. By cultivating mindfulness and awareness during yoga practice, seniors can develop a greater understanding of their physical and emotional needs, empowering them to make informed choices about their health and well-being. With consistent practice and a supportive community, yoga becomes not just a physical exercise but a positive journey toward holistic health and vitality. As seniors embrace the principles of yoga, they discover new levels of resilience, inner strength, and vitality, enabling them to navigate the challenges of aging with grace and equanimity. Please remember always to consult a professional trainer or physician to seek their guidance if you have concerns about yoga.

Yoga offers valuable techniques for managing pain and addressing chronic conditions commonly experienced by seniors. In this chapter, we explore how yoga can be adapted to alleviate discomfort, improve mobility, and enhance overall well-being in seniors facing various health challenges.

One of the key benefits of yoga for pain management is its emphasis on gentle movement, breath awareness, and mindfulness. Seniors with chronic pain conditions such as arthritis, fibromyalgia, or lower back pain can benefit from practicing yoga poses that promote flexibility, strength, and relaxation.

For individuals with arthritis:

- Gentle yoga poses that focus on increasing joint mobility and reducing inflammation can provide relief from stiffness and discomfort.
- Poses such as the Cat-Cow stretch, gentle spinal twists, and child's

pose help lubricate the joints, improve flexibility, and alleviate tension in the muscles surrounding the affected areas.

Seniors with fibromyalgia:

- Seniors can benefit from the gentle stretching and relaxation techniques inherent in yoga practice.
- Restorative yoga poses such as Legs-Up-The-Wall, Supported Bridge, and Corpse Pose promote deep relaxation, reduce muscle tension, and calm the nervous system, helping to alleviate the widespread pain and fatigue associated with fibromyalgia.

Seniors dealing with lower back pain:

- Yoga poses that strengthen the core muscles, improve posture, and increase spinal flexibility can offer significant relief.
- Poses such as Cobra Pose, Cat-Cow stretch, and Supine Twist help lengthen and strengthen the back muscles, release tension in the spine, and improve overall spinal health.

In addition to physical pain, yoga can help seniors manage chronic conditions such as hypertension, diabetes, and cardiovascular disease by promoting relaxation, reducing stress, and improving circulation. Practices like gentle yoga sequences, deep breathing exercises, and meditation can help seniors regulate blood pressure, balance blood sugar levels, and support heart health.

Yoga also offers valuable tools for managing stress, anxiety, and depression, which often accompany chronic pain and illness. Mindfulness-based practices such as guided meditation, body scan, and loving-kindness meditation help seniors cultivate resilience, emotional balance, and a sense of inner peace in the face of life's challenges.

By incorporating yoga into their daily routines, seniors can develop greater self-awareness, cultivate a deeper connection to their bodies, and learn effective strategies for managing pain and chronic conditions. With regular practice and guidance from qualified instructors, yoga can become a powerful tool for promoting health, well-being, and vitality at any age. While my parents certainly do not classify themselves as yoga professionals, they sure have enjoyed the journey of improved health and wellness.

6

Building Strength and Balance with Chair Yoga

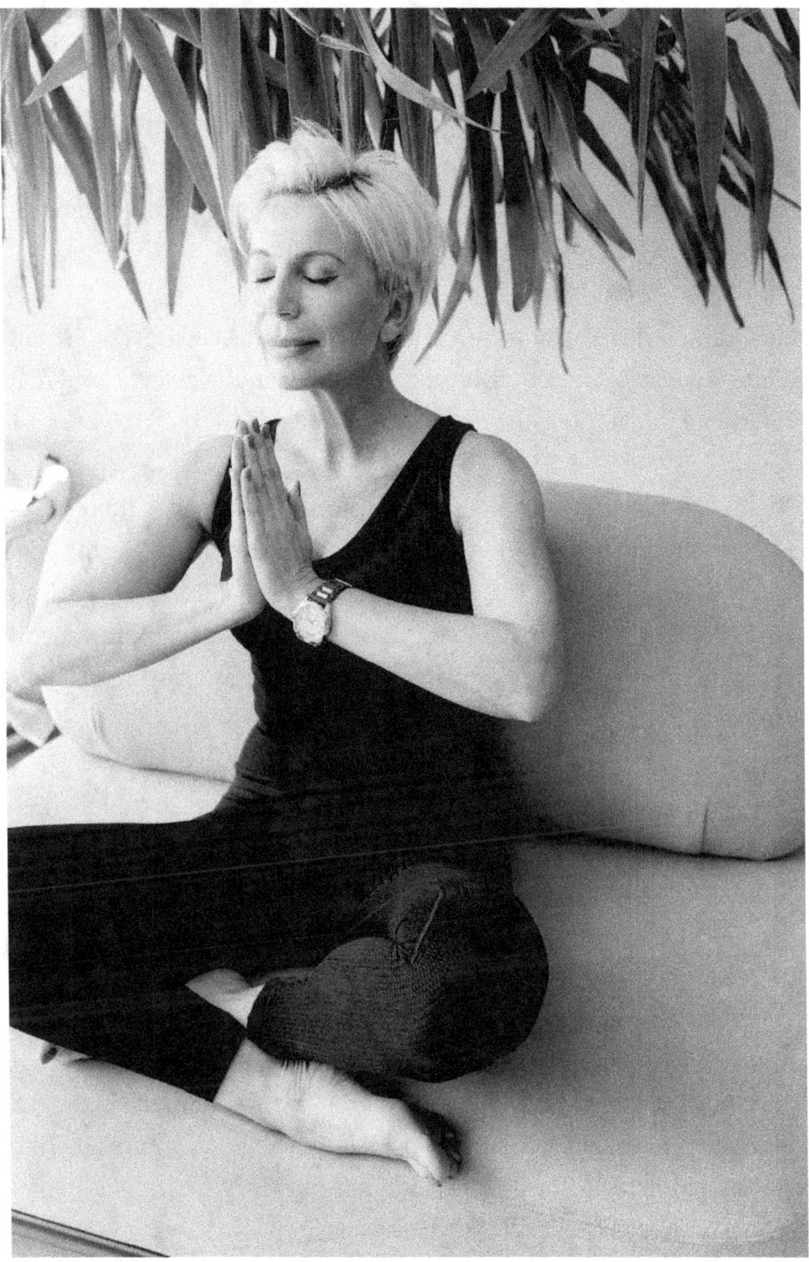

I n addition to the physical benefits, chair yoga offers seniors profound mental and emotional advantages. The practice emphasizes mindfulness, which involves paying attention to the present moment without judgment. Seniors can cultivate a deeper connection to themselves and their surroundings through mindful awareness of both the body and breath.

I have also written a book specifically about Chair Exercises for Seniors. While it doesn't fully describe yoga exercises in the chair, it will help guide you.

Chair yoga encourages seniors to become more attuned to their sensations, thoughts, and emotions. By practicing mindfulness during yoga poses, seniors can develop greater self-awareness and acceptance, leading to reduced stress, anxiety, and depression. The gentle movements and focused breathing of chair yoga promote relaxation, calmness, and a sense of inner peace.

The meditative aspect of chair yoga encourages seniors to explore their inner landscape and develop resilience in facing life's challenges. By integrating mindfulness and meditation into their practice, seniors can cultivate greater emotional balance, resilience, and well-being, empowering them to navigate the ups and downs of aging with grace and calmness.

Chair yoga offers seniors a safe and effective way to build strength, improve balance, and enhance overall well-being. Make sure you find yourself the right chair that is comfortable for you. Whether you're new to yoga or have limited mobility, chair yoga provides accessible options to experience the benefits of this ancient practice. Here are some key elements and poses to help you build strength and balance through chair yoga:

Seated Mountain Pose (Tadasana):

- Begin by sitting tall in your chair with your feet flat on the ground and your spine straight.
- Ground your feet into the floor, engage your core muscles, and roll your shoulders back and down.
- Lift the crown of your head towards the ceiling, lengthening your spine.
- This pose helps improve posture and stability while promoting a sense of grounding and centering.

Seated Warrior Pose (Virabhadrasana):

- Extend one leg forward from the seated mountain pose and place your foot firmly on the ground.
- Keep your other foot grounded and stable.
- Raise your arms overhead, stretching them towards the sky.
- Engage your core muscles and lengthen through your spine.
- This pose strengthens the legs, improves balance, and increases focus and concentration.

Seated Forward Bend (Paschimottanasana):

- Sit towards the front of your chair with your feet flat on the floor and hip-width apart.
- Inhale to lengthen your spine, then exhale as you hinge forward from your hips, leading with your chest.
- Depending on your flexibility, allow your hands to rest on your thighs or shins.

- Keep your neck relaxed and gaze forward.
- This pose stretches the spine, hamstrings, and lower back while calming the mind and reducing stress.

Seated Twist (Ardha Matsyendrasana):

- Sit towards the front of your chair with your feet flat on the floor and your spine tall.
- Place your right hand on the back of the chair and your left hand on your right knee.
- Inhale to lengthen your spine, then exhale as you gently twist to the right, using your hands for support.
- Keep your shoulders relaxed and your gaze soft. Hold the twist for a few breaths, then repeat on the other side.
- Twists improve spinal mobility, aid digestion, and stimulate detoxification.

Incorporating these chair yoga poses into your daily routine can help you build strength, improve balance, and support overall physical and mental well-being. Remember to listen to your body and practice mindfulness while exploring the movements. With consistency and patience, chair yoga can become a valuable tool for promoting health, vitality, and longevity in your senior years.

7

Creating a Personalized Yoga Practice

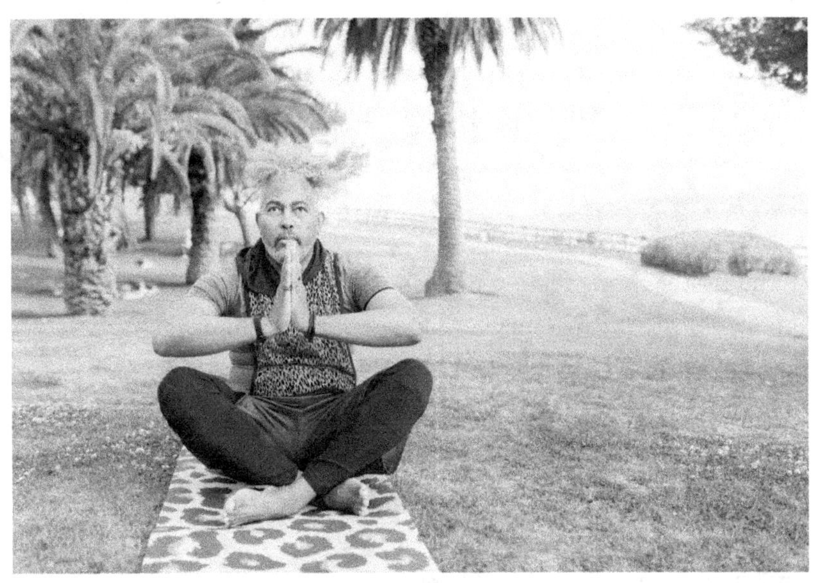

Additionally, seniors should keep a yoga journal to track their progress, experiences, and reflections. This journal can serve as a valuable tool for self-discovery and growth, allowing seniors to observe patterns, set intentions, and celebrate achievements along their yoga journey. Regularly reviewing the journal can provide insight into the effectiveness of the practice and help seniors stay motivated and committed to their wellness goals.

Moreover, practicing yoga with a supportive community or joining yoga classes tailored for seniors can foster a sense of connection, camaraderie, and encouragement, enhancing the overall yoga experience and promoting a sense of belonging and community among practitioners.

For those go-getters, creating a personalized yoga practice allows seniors to tailor their yoga experience to meet their unique needs, preferences, and goals. By customizing their practice, seniors can maximize the benefits of yoga while ensuring that it aligns with their physical abilities and limitations.

Assessing Individual Needs:

The first step in creating a personalized yoga practice is to assess individual needs and considerations. Seniors should consider their current fitness level, health conditions, mobility restrictions, and personal goals. Consulting with a healthcare provider or a certified yoga instructor can provide valuable insights and guidance in developing a safe and effective practice.

Choosing Appropriate Yoga Styles:

Seniors have a variety of yoga styles to choose from, each offering distinct benefits and approaches. Hatha, gentle, chair, restorative, and yin yoga are particularly well-suited for seniors due to their emphasis on gentle movements, relaxation, and breath awareness. Seniors can explore different styles to find the one that resonates most with their preferences and needs.

Selecting Suitable Yoga Poses:

Once the yoga style is chosen, seniors can select specific yoga poses that address their areas of focus and concern. For example, seniors looking to improve flexibility may incorporate a variety of stretching poses, while those focusing on strength may include more standing or balance poses. Chair yoga poses can be modified and adapted to accommodate varying levels of mobility and flexibility.

Establishing a Consistent Routine:

Consistency is key to reaping the benefits of yoga. Seniors should establish a regular practice schedule that suits their lifestyle and commitments. Starting with short, manageable sessions and gradually increasing the duration and intensity can help seniors build stamina and progress safely over time.

Listening to the Body:

Seniors should listen to their bodies throughout the practice and honor their limitations. It's essential to practice mindfulness and self-awareness, noticing any signs of discomfort, strain, or fatigue. Seniors should modify poses as needed, use props for support and stability, and take breaks when necessary to prevent injury and promote overall well-being.

Incorporating Breath-work and Meditation:

Breathwork and meditation are integral components of yoga that can enhance relaxation, focus, and inner peace. Seniors can incorporate gentle breathing exercises, guided meditation, and mindfulness techniques into their practice to promote mental clarity, reduce stress, and cultivate a sense of calmness and well-being. I know my parents often use breathing exercises when they're feeling anxious or stressed.

By creating a personalized yoga practice, seniors can experience the positive effects of yoga while honoring their bodies and individual needs. A tailored yoga practice empowers seniors to embark on a journey of self-discovery, healing, and holistic well-being, fostering vitality, joy, and resilience in their lives.

8

Overcoming Challenges and Obstacles

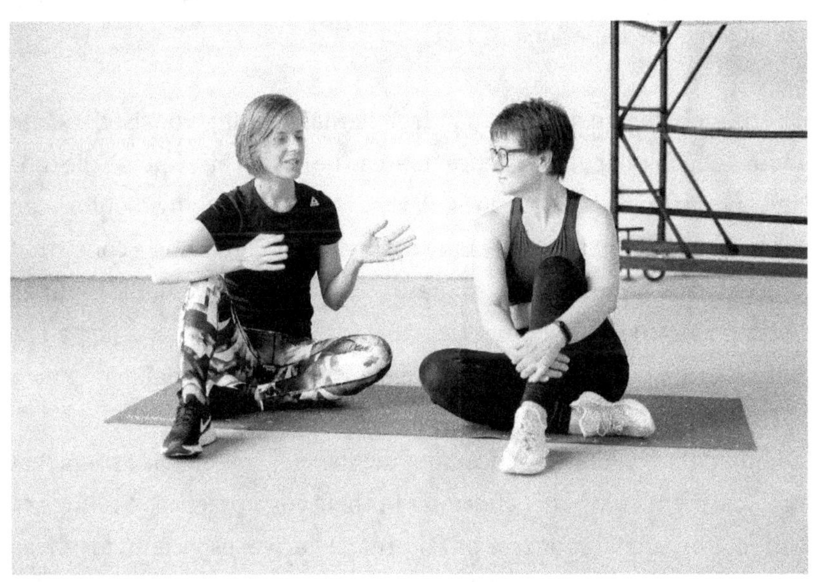

As seniors embark on their yoga journey, they may encounter various challenges and obstacles along the way. However, with patience, perseverance, and the right mindset, these challenges can be overcome, allowing seniors to reap the full benefits of their yoga practice.

One common challenge for seniors is physical limitations or pre-existing health conditions that may affect their ability to perform certain yoga poses. It's essential for seniors to listen to their bodies and modify poses as needed to accommodate their individual needs and limitations. Yoga instructors specializing in senior yoga can offer valuable guidance and support, providing modifications and alternative poses to ensure a safe and accessible practice for all participants. Please take the extra steps to consult a professional trainer or physician should you have any concerns about yoga participation.

Another challenge seniors may face is maintaining consistency and motivation in their yoga practice. Life can be hectic, and finding the time and energy to practice yoga regularly can be challenging. Seniors can overcome this obstacle by setting realistic goals, creating a consistent practice schedule, and incorporating yoga into their daily routines. Setting aside dedicated time each day for yoga, even if it's just a few minutes, can help cultivate consistency and establish a habit.

Additionally, seniors may encounter mental and emotional barriers that prevent them from fully engaging in their yoga practice. Feelings of self-doubt, anxiety, or fear of failure may arise, especially for those who are new to yoga or have limited experience with physical activity. Seniors must cultivate self-compassion, patience, and an open mind as they navigate these challenges. Yoga is a practice of self-discovery and self-acceptance, and embracing imperfection and progress at their own pace is okay.

Seniors may also face external obstacles such as financial constraints, lack of access to yoga classes, or limited social support. Fortunately, many resources are available to help overcome these challenges. Seniors can explore free or low-cost yoga classes in their community, access online yoga tutorials and resources, or seek out community centers or senior organizations that offer yoga programs tailored for older adults.

Additionally, connecting with like-minded individuals and building a support network of fellow yoga practitioners can provide encouragement, accountability, and motivation to overcome obstacles and stay committed to their practice. My parents love doing yoga in the comfort of their home in front of the television. There are so many options to practice yoga virtually, either free or low-cost.

In conclusion, while seniors may encounter various challenges and obstacles on their yoga journey, each obstacle presents an opportunity for growth, learning, and transformation. By approaching challenges with resilience, determination, and an open heart, seniors can overcome barriers, deepen their yoga practice, and experience profound physical, mental, and emotional benefits that support their overall health and well-being.

9

Yoga for Healthy Aging and Longevity

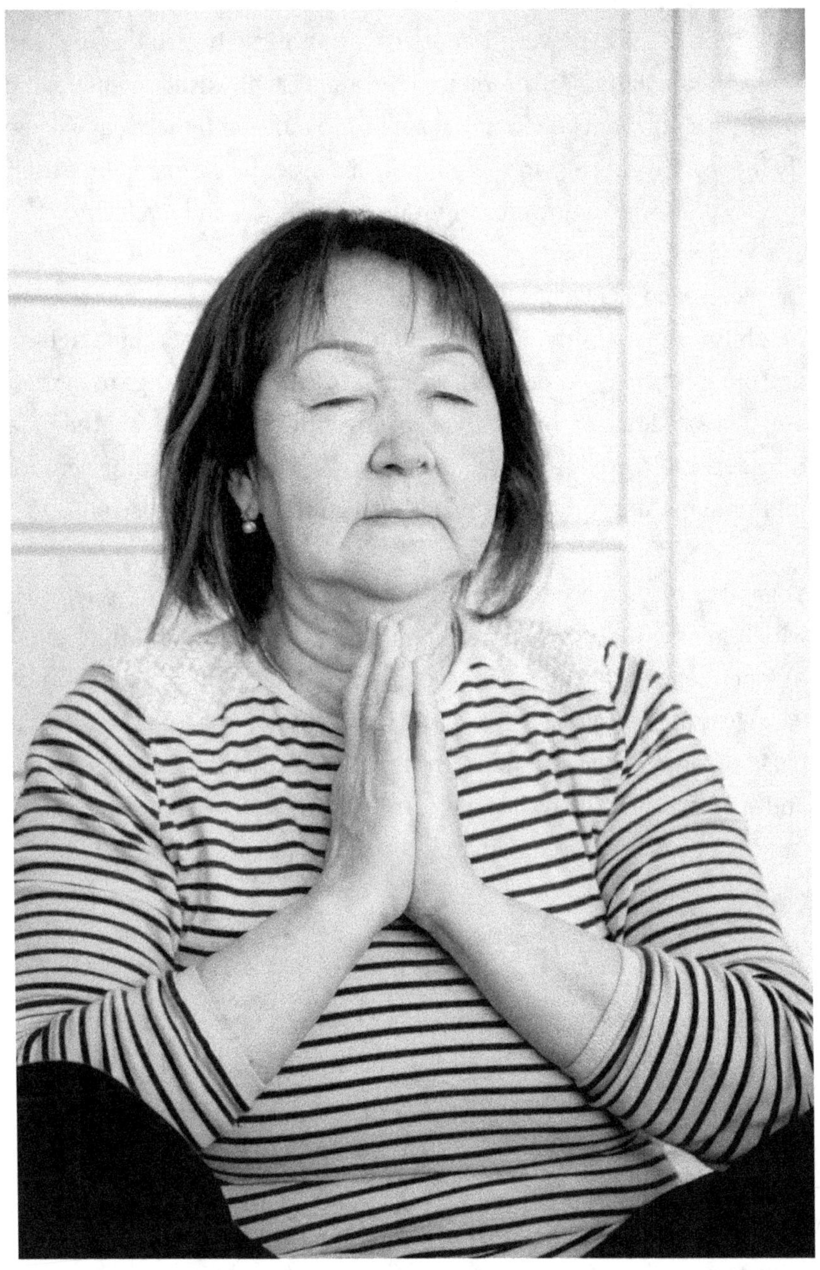

Yoga is a powerful tool for promoting healthy aging and longevity. It offers a wide range of physical, mental, and emotional benefits that support overall well-being as we age. By incorporating yoga into their daily lives, seniors can enhance their quality of life and enjoy greater vitality, resilience, and longevity.

One key benefit of yoga for healthy aging is its ability to promote flexibility and mobility. As we age, our muscles tend to become tighter, and our joints may become stiff, leading to a decreased range of motion and increased risk of injury. Yoga poses gently stretch and lengthen the muscles, lubricate the joints, and improve flexibility, helping seniors maintain mobility and prevent age-related stiffness and discomfort.

Yoga also plays a crucial role in building strength and muscle tone, which is essential for maintaining balance, stability, and functional independence as we age. Many yoga poses require the engagement of various muscle groups, helping to strengthen the core, legs, arms, and back. Strong muscles support proper posture, reduce the risk of falls, and enhance overall physical performance, allowing seniors to engage fully in daily activities and maintain an active lifestyle.

In addition to physical benefits, yoga offers numerous mental and emotional advantages for healthy aging. Yoga practices such as mindfulness meditation and conscious breathing help seniors cultivate a calm, centered mind, reduce stress, and promote emotional resilience. By learning to be present at the moment and let go of worries and distractions, seniors can experience greater peace, contentment, and mental clarity, enhancing their overall quality of life.

Furthermore, yoga fosters a sense of connection and community, which is vital for healthy aging. Practicing yoga in a group setting allows seniors to connect with like-minded individuals, share experiences, and build meaningful relationships. The sense of camaraderie and support that arises from practicing yoga together creates a positive and uplifting environment that nourishes the spirit and promotes social engagement and well-being.

Another significant benefit of yoga for healthy aging is its ability to promote heart health and overall cardiovascular fitness. Yoga practices such as gentle flow sequences and breath-centered movements help improve circulation, lower blood pressure and reduce the risk of heart disease and stroke. By supporting cardiovascular health, yoga contributes to greater vitality, energy, and longevity, allowing seniors to lead active and fulfilling lives well into their later years.

In conclusion, yoga offers a holistic approach to healthy aging, addressing the physical, mental, emotional, and social aspects of well-being. By embracing yoga as a lifelong practice, seniors can enjoy improved flexibility, strength, balance, mental clarity, and heart health, leading to greater longevity and vitality as they age. With dedication, consistency, and an open heart, yoga can become a powerful ally in the journey toward healthy aging and a fulfilling life.

10

Integrating Yoga into Daily Life

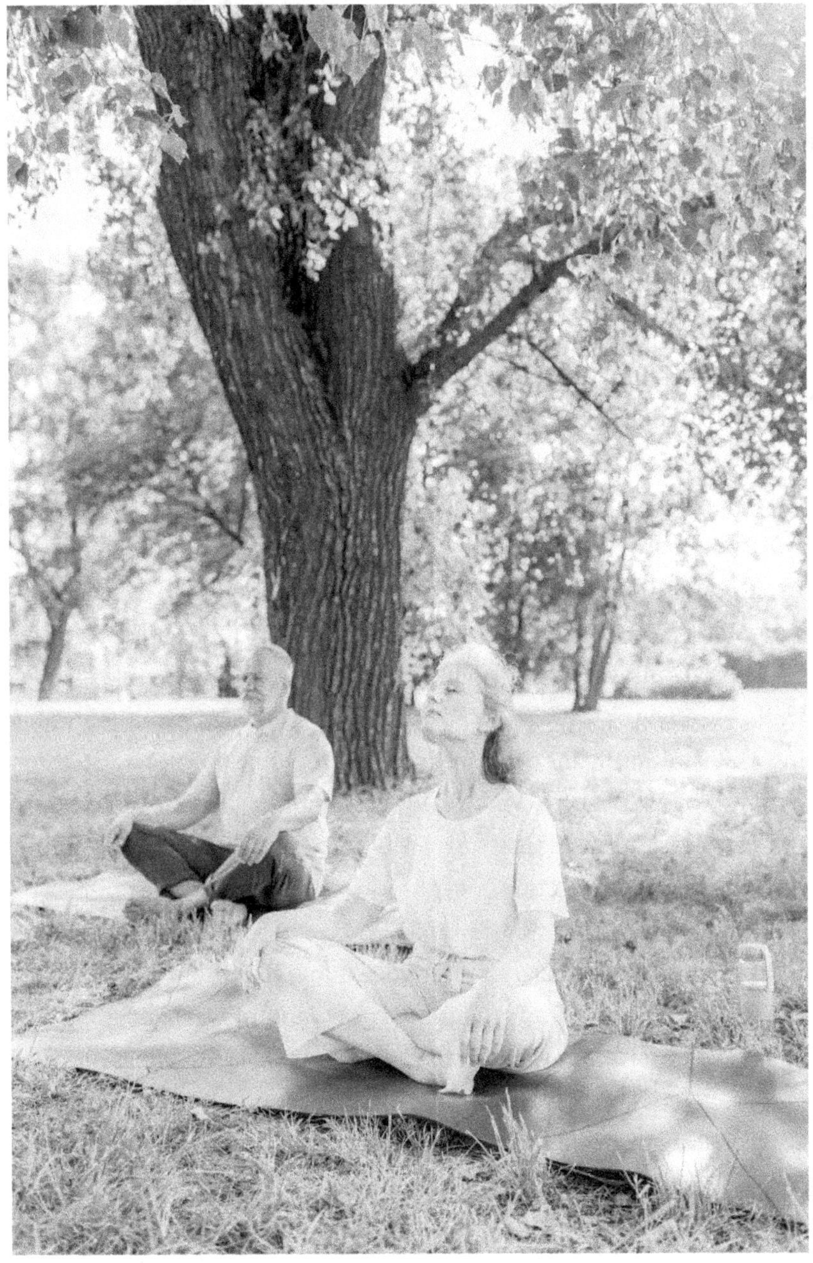

Integrating yoga into daily life is key to experiencing its full benefits and making it a sustainable practice for seniors. By incorporating yoga into various aspects of daily routines, seniors can cultivate mindfulness, promote physical health, and enhance overall well-being.

One way to integrate yoga into daily life is by establishing a consistent practice schedule. Designate specific times during the day for yoga practice, whether in the morning to energize and set a positive tone, during lunch breaks to alleviate stress and tension, or in the evening to unwind and relax before bedtime. Consistency is key to building a regular yoga habit and reaping its rewards. It's also important to ensure your environment for practicing yoga is comfortable.

In addition to dedicated practice sessions, seniors can weave yoga into everyday activities. They can incorporate mindful breathing exercises while performing household chores, such as deep inhales and exhales while sweeping or washing dishes. They can also practice gentle stretching while waiting in line or sitting at a desk, focusing on releasing tension and improving posture. By infusing mindfulness and movement into mundane tasks, seniors can turn ordinary moments into opportunities for self-care and reflection.

Furthermore, seniors can integrate yoga into social interactions by practicing with friends, family members, or community groups. Joining a yoga class or forming a small group of like-minded individuals provides shared experiences, mutual support, and accountability opportunities. Participating in group yoga sessions fosters a sense of community and connection, enhancing the overall enjoyment and motivation to sustain a yoga practice.

Mindfulness is a central aspect of yoga that can be integrated into various aspects of daily life. Seniors can cultivate mindfulness during every day activities by bringing awareness to sensations, thoughts, and emotions as they arise. Practice mindful eating by savoring each bite, noticing flavors, textures, and aromas, and appreciating the nourishment provided by food. Engage in mindful walking by paying attention to each step, the sensation of the ground beneath your feet, and the sights and sounds around you.

Moreover, seniors can integrate yoga philosophy and principles into decision-making processes and interpersonal relationships. They can apply the yogic principles of compassion, nonjudgment, and acceptance in interactions with others, fostering empathy, understanding, and connection. They can also use mindfulness techniques to manage stress, regulate emotions, and cultivate a sense of inner peace and resilience in the face of challenges.

By integrating yoga into daily life, seniors can experience its transformative effects on physical health, mental well-being, and overall quality of life. Through consistent practice, mindfulness, and intention, yoga becomes more than just a set of poses—it becomes a way of living fully and authentically, enriching every moment with presence, purpose, and joy.

11

Conclusion

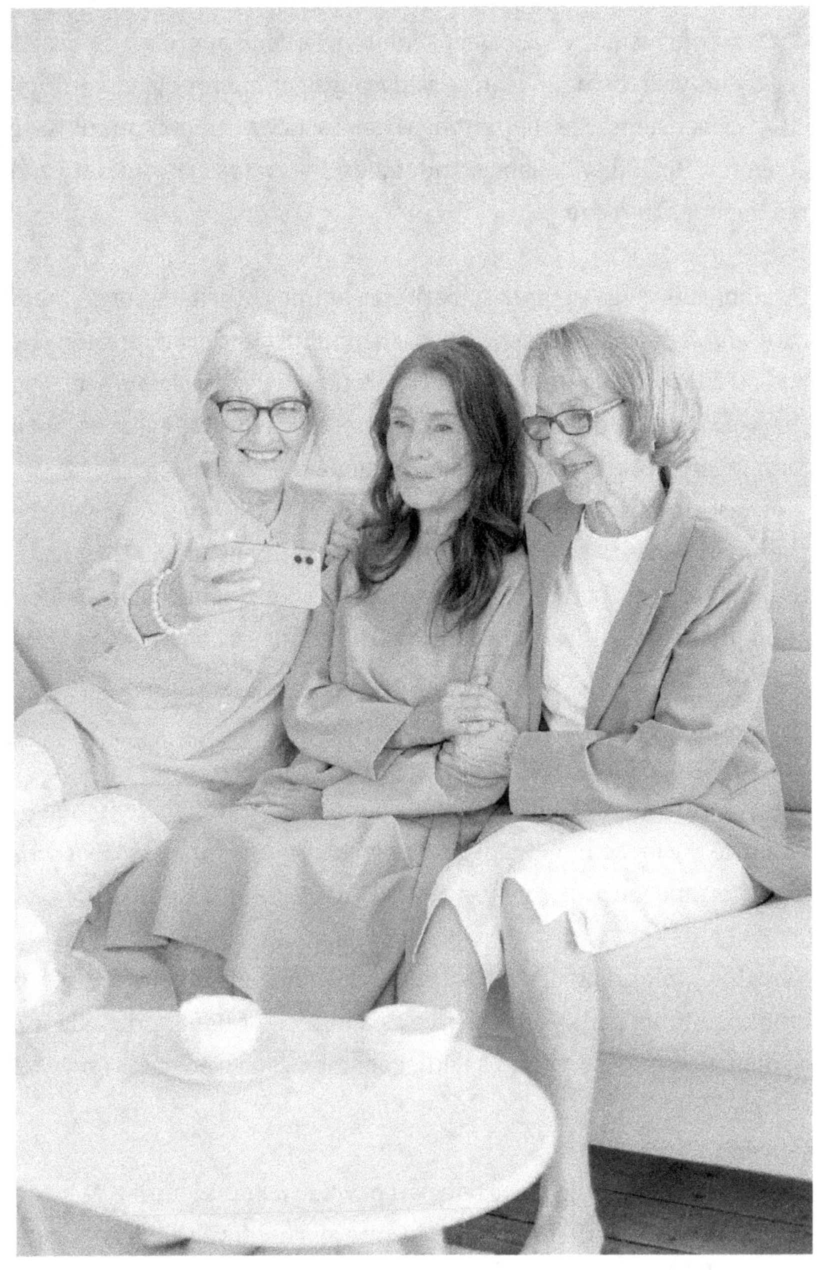

In conclusion, yoga offers seniors a holistic approach to health and well-being, encompassing physical, mental, and spiritual dimensions. Through gentle yoga practices, seniors can cultivate strength, flexibility, balance, and mindfulness, fostering vitality and resilience as they age.

By embracing yoga, seniors embark on a journey of self-discovery, self-care, and self-empowerment. Through mindful movement, breathwork, and meditation, they deepen their connection to themselves, others, and the world around them. Yoga becomes not just a form of exercise, but a path to inner peace, clarity, and fulfillment.

As seniors integrate yoga into their daily lives, they discover the profound benefits of living mindfully and authentically. They learn to listen to their bodies, honor their limitations, and celebrate their strengths. They cultivate gratitude for the gift of each moment and find joy in life's simple pleasures.

Ultimately, yoga is a practice of transformation and renewal—a journey of awakening to the fullness of life's possibilities. It is an invitation to embrace the present moment with open hearts and minds, to live with intention and purpose, and to age gracefully and with dignity.

May this exploration of yoga for seniors inspire and empower all who embark on this path. May it serve as a beacon of light and guidance, illuminating the way toward health, happiness, and wholeness for years to come

Thank you for allowing me to be a part of your wellness journey. May the insights gained within these pages inspire and uplift you as you navigate the beautiful tapestry of life.

I sincerely hope you had as much fun reading this book as I did writing it! If you enjoyed it, please take the time to give me a favorable review on Amazon. The success of my writing journey is an outcome of positive experiences. Thank you!

Here's to a future filled with flexibility, strength, and balance - in body, mind, and spirit."

N.L. Cash

12

Resources

References:

R

- McCall, T. (2007). Yoga as Medicine: The Yogic Prescription for Health and Healing. Bantam.
- Saraswati, S. S. (2000). Asana Pranayama Mudra Bandha. Yoga Publications Trust.
- McCall, T. (2010). Yoga Journal's Yoga for Health: The Healing Art of Yoga Therapy. Random House LLC.
- Iyengar, B. K. S. (1979). Light on Yoga: Yoga Dipika. Schocken.
- Mehta, S., Mehta, M., & Mehta, S. (1990). Yoga: The Iyengar Way. Dorling Kindersley.
- Birch, B. (2006). Power Yoga: The Total Strength and Flexibility Workout. Simon and Schuster.
- Kabat-Zinn, J. (1994). Wherever You Go, There You Are: Mindfulness Meditation in Everyday Life. Hyperion.
- Salzberg, S. (2011). Real Happiness: The Power of Meditation: A 28-Day Program. Workman Publishing.
- Goldstein, J., & Kornfield, J. (2001). Seeking the Heart of

Wisdom: The Path of Insight Meditation. Shambhala.

· Fishman, L., & Saltonstall, E. (2011). Yoga for Arthritis: The Complete Guide. Shambhala.

· Cushman, A. (2004). Moving into Stillness: A Practical Guide to Qigong and Meditation. Shambhala.

· Walshe, M. (2007). The Longevity Bible: 8 Essential Strategies for Keeping Your Mind Sharp and Your Body Young. Rodale Books.

· Lakshmi Voelker Chair Yoga. (n.d.). Retrieved from https://www.getfitwhereyousit.com/

· Lakshmi Voelker Chair Yoga: Seated Yoga for the Health of It. (n.d.). Retrieved from https://www.getfitwhereyousit.com/

· Los Angeles Public Library. (n.d.). Chair Yoga. Retrieved from https://www.lapl.org/branches/central-library/chair-yoga

· Swami Satyananda Saraswati. (2013). Asana Pranayama Mudra Bandha/2008 Fourth Revised Edition. Bihar School of Yoga.

· Feuerstein, G. (2012). The Yoga Tradition: Its History, Literature, Philosophy, and Practice. Hohm Press.

· Farhi, D. (2000). Yoga Mind, Body & Spirit: A Return to Wholeness. Holt Paperbacks.

· Sears, W. (2012). Yoga for Body, Breath, and Mind: A Guide to Personal Reintegration. Simon and Schuster.

· Robinson, T. (2011). The Yoga Bible. Walking Stick Press.

· Smith, J. (2013). The Complete Guide to Yin Yoga: The Philosophy and Practice of Yin Yoga. Lotus Publishing.

· McCall, T. (2016). Yoga for Healthy Aging: A Guide to Lifelong Well-Being. Shambhala.

· AARP. (n.d.). Health and Wellness: Yoga. Retrieved from

https://www.aarp.org/health/fitness/yoga/

- Stephenson, S. (2002). Yoga on the Ball: Enhance Your Yoga Practice Using the Exercise Ball. Inner Traditions.
- Hayes, M., & Stein, K. (2010). The Everything Guide to Yoga: Pose, Postures, Breathing Exercises, Meditation, and Guidance for Health and Well-Being. Simon and Schuster.
- Hirschkorn, E. (2013). Yoga for Dummies. Wiley Publishing.
- Sovik, R. (2000). Yoga: Mastering the Basics. Himalayan Institute Press.
- Kaminoff, L., & Matthews, A. (2012). Yoga Anatomy. Human Kinetics.
- Lasater, J. (1995). Relax and Renew: Restful Yoga for Stressful Times. Rodmell Press.
- Yee, R., & Stiles, T. (2006). Yoga: The Poetry of the Body. Rodale Books.
- U.S. Census Bureau
- Pexels.com